Boost Your
Weight Loss
with Acupressure

Anne Cossé

"Boost your Weight Loss with Acupressure"
December 2014
ISBN 979-10-92669-03-9

Also by Anne Cossé:

"Facial Rejuvenation Acupressure, Look 10 Years Younger in 10 Min per Day"
Paperback, Kindle, PDF. Visit www.acupressurewellness.com

The information provided in this tutorial is for educational and informational purposes only and in no way should be considered as an offering of medical advice. This information should not replace consultation with a competent healthcare professional. The reader should regularly consult a licensed health care professional in matters relating to their weight and health, and particularly in respect to any symptoms that may require diagnosis or medical attention. The author is in no way liable for any misuse of the material.

Please note that the author cannot provide personal email consultancy to readers. Thank you for your understanding!

Table of Contents

Foreword

So you bought the book (thank you). But you might still be wondering: can I really rub a few spots somewhere on my body and make my urge to overeat disappear? Can I apply pressure with my fingers and... lose weight?

It sounds too good to be true, I know.

Yet there is so much clinical and empirical evidence that acupressure is effective—for stress reduction, pain relief, labor induction and more—that it is now being used at top medical centers and universities around the world. Including Yale and Johns Hopkins! And they are seeing weight-loss patients get great results.

Like so many people, perhaps you have tried to make healthier choices in the past and did not see much difference on the scale. Good news: acupressure can really give you that extra boost you are looking for.

Dieting alone is not enough as an effective weight-loss program. Shifting to a diet with less carbs, more proteins and more fiber is excellent for temporarily losing weight, but it does not get at the causes of food addictions, obsessions, yearnings and cravings. People can lose weight on low-calorie or low-carb diets, but that kind of diet change is not a deep shift, so they tend to gain it back.

Adding acupressure to your weight loss program (healthy food, exercise, etc) can make it work better *and* help maintaining your initial weight loss afterwards.

Clinical research shows that:
- acupressure techniques make an ordinary diet work a whopping 300% better
- acupressure cures cravings completely for 89% of people

- most acupressure techniques help lower levels of belly-fattening stress hormones

The Western research has discovered that the meridians described in Traditional Chinese Medicine actually correspond to areas of the body where nerve centers, blood vessels muscles and intricate webs of connective tissue converge to form powerful pathways to the brain. So when scientists stimulate points traditionally thought to improve mood, for example, MRI studies are showing increased production of feel-good brain chemicals, such as dopamine and serotonin.

That is why acupressure is a great booster for weight loss: it works on the underlying causes of your weight issues, like stress.

Other studies have shown that stimulating traditional hunger-control acupressure / acupuncture points prompts the brain's appetite center to produce stop-eating hormones. That's an additional level on which acupressure operates.

While research to determine the exact mechanisms that make acupressure work is still in its early stages, we know for sure that there is zero risk of side effects. There is no harm in trying it—and there are tremendous benefits. Plus, it is easy to do, can be used anywhere—and it's free!

Now some important words about dieting....

I share the following opinion about dieting: do NOT diet by drastically reducing your calories intake!

If you reside in the USA you might be shocked by that statement, because in the USA weight control is all about calories. But the truth of the matter is that very low calorie dieting may result in quick weight loss but it almost always results in lowering your metabolism - and that change tends to stay with you long after the diet is history.
Furthermore, depriving your metabolism of calories is a sure way to dive in a spiral of fatigue (no fuel for the body) and moodiness.

Calories are not the main culprits. Carbs, grease and stress are.

So, how do you go about making a permanent change in your weight?

1 - Don't starve yourself.

2 - Increase your fiber intake.

A study published in the October 17, 1999, issue of the Journal of the American Medical Association (JAMA), reported that one of the best ways to control your weight is to increase your dietary fiber. Fiber helps you to feel full without adding much food. And certain kinds of fiber, such as psyllium husks, have the ability to absorb fat from the foods we eat, carrying that fat out of the body before it is absorbed. That's how 'fat grabbers' work. Additionally, fiber has been shown to help lower serum cholesterol, reduce risk for cancer, and help diabetics control their blood sugar levels better.

3 - Cleanse.

It is generally recommended that all weight reduction programs begin with a thorough cleansing program. Modern food processing removes most of the enzymes and fiber from our foods. And the staples of our diet - meat and dairy products - contain no fiber at all. Inadequate fiber slows the movement of the intestines and encourages the buildup of waste and toxins in the bowel, liver and blood. Accumulated toxins have been linked with diverse health problems including fibromyalgia, cancer, Irritable Bowel Syndrome (IBS), poor skin, headaches, high blood pressure and digestive disturbances. Everyone can benefit from a periodic cleanse to clear out these accumulations.
However, be gentle with yourself: you don't have to go overboard in that field.

4 - Eat well.

Eat at least 5 servings of vegetables and fruit each day. They are full of vitamins, minerals and other phytonutrients as well as fiber. Include lean protein, a variety of beans, whole grains, raw nuts and seeds.

Minimize high fat foods - these come mostly from snack foods (potato chips, cookies, and highly processed foods) and cheese. Increasing your protein and reducing the carbohydrates in your diet has shown to be effective to many people.

Note that it is all about dosage: increase or decrease, but do not eliminate completely. Except highly processed food. Try to eat organic, natural food as much as you can.

5 - Drink plenty of water.

Don't worry, it will not result in weight gain! "Plenty of water" means enough to help fiber to move out the toxins and your kidneys to flush them out. There are different rules circulating, I find all of them unrealistic and definitely too rigid. If you don't go often and/or if your pee is darkish and/or if you feel tension in your head (like a headache), you don't drink enough. It's that simple.

Important: drink *water*. Coffee, fruit juice, tea, herbal tea are not water. Would you wash your hair or windows with those? That's what I thought... The inside of your body is no different.

6 - Exercise 30 minutes three times a week.

It is not about becoming an athlete and hitting the gym every day; it is about moving it on and enjoying it. For instance, walk as much as possible. It will stimulate your metabolism and you really will feel better, have more energy, and ultimately lose weight.

7- Use acupressure every day.

Acupressure regulates hunger, digestion, hormones and stress (more on that in Part 3 of this book). That's how the real shift can take place.

Module 1:

Understanding Acupressure

What is acupressure?

How does acupressure work?

Is acupressure safe?

Acupressure Vs western medicine

What is acupressure?

Acupressure is a **natural therapy** where the therapist uses gentle to firm finger pressure (as well as the fist, elbow or feet) to stimulate the energy flow in the body, strengthen its self-healing capabilities and enable it to fend off illness better.

Acupressure is one of the three main branches of Traditional Chinese Medicine and is similar to acupuncture except that here the therapist applies pressure to specific pressure points in the body with natural means rather than needles.
Acupressure is often confused with massage, which is quite simplistic by comparison.

The origins of acupressure are as ancient as the instinctive impulse to hold your forehead or temples when you have a headache. Everyone at one time or another has used his/her hands to hold tense or painful places on the body.

More than 5,000 years ago, the Chinese discovered that by pressing certain points on the body, the pain in that pressure point could be relieved. They also found this application of pressure to benefit other parts of the body further away from the pain point.

Gradually, they identified several pressure points that not only alleviated pain but also influenced the functioning of certain internal organs.
A growing number of data and scientific studies show why and how acupuncture and acupressure are efficient, and more and more studies explain and validate the efficiency of this natural healing art.

Acupressure helps to:
- Strengthen the **vital energy**
- Relieve **physical pain**
- Soothe **muscular tension**
- Boost the **immune system**
- Regulate the **mood and emotions**

To know more about the many benefits of acupressure, visit
www.annecosse.com

How does acupressure work?

Acupressure follows the 5,000 year old concepts of Traditional Chinese Medicine.

The vital energy

Eastern tradition describes the world in terms of **energy**. Energy is the elementary substance and vital life force. It is also a synonym of "breath". The Qi evokes breath, movement and vital energy. It encompasses two complimentary aspects: the Yin and the Yang. Without energy, there is no life. All living beings have this energy. It goes way beyond simple muscular energy. It encompasses all the energies a body can pull: **physical, mental, physiological and psychological.**

This flow is called Qi or Ch'i in Chinese (as in Qi Gong and Tai Chi Chuan), Ki in Japanese (as in Aikido) and Prana in India. In the West it is referred to by scientists as bio-electricity and as orgone by Dr W. Reich.

According to traditional Chinese medicine, the Qi is always moving. Ancient Chinese doctors observed that the health of every person depends on the **good circulation** of the vital energy in the body, and on its two polarities, the Yin and the Yang.

The meridians

In the same way that blood is transported by veins, vital energy circulates around the body along a network of **subtle paths**: the Meridians.

The Meridians were identified 5,000 years ago in China.
There are **12 main Meridians**. Eleven of these cross a vital organ and are named after it: Lungs, Large Intestine, Stomach, Spleen, Heart, Small Intestine, Bladder, Kidneys, Pericardium, Gall Bladder, Liver. The 12th Meridian, Triple Warmer, does not relate to any organ.
The 12 Meridians partner in 6 pairs of 1 Yin Meridian and 1 Yang Meridian.

Each Meridian continues to operate if the associated organ is removed. This is also true in cases where a limb has been removed. The Chi of the meridians extends to where the limb would naturally end.

At some specific points along the Meridian paths, the Qi is near the skin and thus physically accessible. These points are the famous acupuncture points, or **acupoints** (called tsubos in Japanese). They are the gateways to the Qi, and to the whole energy system. To work on the acupoints, acupuncture uses needles while acupressure uses gentle to firm finger pressure (as well as the fist, elbow or feet, depending on the technique).

Acupoints are particularly sensitive to bio-electricity, and convey it very quickly. That is how modern science proved their existence.
When the Ki does not flow well, some tsubos become too full or too empty, which generates physical and psychological dysfunction.

The 12 main Meridians are linked together by another layer of 8 Extraordinary Channels. This network regulates the Ki between the Meridians, and hence the harmonious interaction between the organs. The Extraordinary Channels do not have their own acupoints, but flow through the points of more than one main Meridian. Some of those "borrowed" points are Master Points: by simply applying enough to pressure to these Master Points, one can regulate the whole Extraordinary Channel to which it belongs.

The Yin and the Yang

Yin and Yang are **the two sides of everything** in the universe. Outsight and insight, hot and cold, day and night, action and rest, hardness and softness, hallow and deep... one cannot exist without the other.
The Chinese symbol of Yin and Yang perfectly shows this opposition/link: the Yin (in black) and the Yang (in white) are distinct, but create one another (circle) and each one carries the germ of the other (small dot of the opposite color).

The Qi, like electricity, can move thanks to 2 opposing poles. Electricity moves between the positive (+) and negative (-) poles. The Qi moves between the Yin and the Yang.

If the Yin and Yang are out of harmony and balance, the Qi does not flow properly (too strong or too weak, for instance).

The 5 Elements

The Ancient Chinese conceived life and the Universe as a constant interaction between the Yin and Yang. They observed these **relationships in nature** and applied them to the **dynamics of the body**.
The 5 elements are the 5 major characteristics that describe this phenomenon: **wood, fire, earth, metal and water**.

Each element is associated with a yin organ, a yang organ, a body tissue, a sense organ, a body fluid, a flavor, an odor, a moment of the day, an activity, a mental ability, an emotion and a voice type.
Example: Wood = liver, gall bladder, ligaments and tendons, eyes, tears, sour, rancid, morning, beginning, planning, control, anger, loud.
Every human being is made up of the five elements, but one predominates.

An indivisible trio: body, mind and emotions

In Chinese medicine, **the body and mind constantly influence each other**. Emotions are ingrained in the body, and physical pain is a condition of the mind.
Our health and harmony depend on the free and regular flowing of vital energy within our body, mind and emotions.

When any stress disrupts this flow, all the spheres of our being are affected. Not only do we yield to fear, anger and sadness, but we are more prone to illnesses. Depression and anxiety may set in. On the contrary, when body and mind are balanced and in harmony with each other, the energy flows freely, we adjust more easily to a range of emotions, and we feel more joy.

Stress-related tension tends to concentrate on the acupoints. Pressure on these points enables the muscle to stretch and relax, freeing the way to the bloodstream. Toxins are released and flushed away. The bloodstream increase enables more oxygen and nutrients to be conveyed to the body and organs. The body becomes more resistant to disease.

Tension and pain find their source in the accumulation and/or the suppression of negative emotions, and in psychological shocks. That is why acupressure is a valuable ally to restore and strengthen our emotional and psychic balance.

Is acupressure safe?

Acupressure **does not involve any intake or mechanical manipulation**. It bears no related side effect, and cannot overwhelm or flood your body.
Its operating mode is to strengthen your body's **own** self-healing capabilities.

In China and in Japan, acupressure is an official medicine. As such, millions of treatments are given every day. In the USA, acupressure has been used since the 1970's. In this country alone, an average of one million injuries caused by medical procedures and drugs side effects are reported in one single year.

Acupressure is safe, when applied or taught by a certified therapist.

However, people experiencing serious medical problems should always consult their doctor before using any alternative therapies. Serious medical conditions include life-threatening diseases, stroke or heart attack, arteriosclerosis, illnesses caused by bacteria, cancer, contagious skin diseases, or sexually transmitted diseases.

Acupressure is **not** used to treat open wounds, scar tissue, varicose veins, or areas of inflammation. If you are experiencing any of these problems, **consult your physician**.

Acupressure Vs western medicine

In the West, natural therapies are not a substitute to western medicine. It is recommended to inform your doctors about your using acupressure, and why not showing them this book?

However, many clinical trials – carried out in the USA, UK, Norway, Sweden, China, Taiwan, India… -, prove the efficiency of acupressure and acupuncture for many health issues: nausea and vomiting, pain, insomnia, etc. In more and more countries, hospitals and practitioners use acupuncture and acupressure to complement chemical treatments.

In the case of severe diseases (cancer...) and ailments (post-surgery...), acupressure is recommended as an efficient complementary therapy to alleviate pains associated with the condition or with the drug taking or procedure. The most spectacular example would be with cancer patients, to help them bear the strong side effects of chemo and radio therapy.

In some cases, acupressure or acupuncture are even the primary techniques used by doctors. For instance, many midwives and doctors now use acupuncture and acupressure to induce labor, and ease labor-related pain.

Another common ailment that can be treated with acupressure is lower back pain.

Should you or your physicians have any queries about acupressure and acupuncture efficiency, clinical trials and studies' conclusions are available on http://nccam.nih.gov, a service of the U.S. Department of Health and the National Institutes of Health.

Module 2:

Guidelines to Practicing Self-Acupressure

How do I locate the points?

How do I work on the points?

How much pressure should I apply?

What else should I do?

How do I locate the points?

The practical way to locate the acupoints on your body is to use **anatomical landmarks.** That is how practitioners can find the points on their patients' body, even though bodies come in so many forms and shapes!

Anatomical landmarks are mainly the bone indentations and protrusions, but also creases and articulations, muscles joints and cords, and miscellaneous elements such as the navel, the eye brows...

All the points in this book are illustrated with a description of these landmarks, in addition of pictures.

If you need to refer to a chart to locate a point, here is the way to go. Each point is assigned an **identification number** to track its placement along the body. It is made of the meridian name initial, and the sequence order of that point along the meridian. For instance: K3 = 3rd point on the Kidneys meridian), GB41 = 41th point on the Gall Bladder meridian.

This is the standard referencing system used by professional acupressurists and acupuncturists around the world.

You do NOT need to know or remember any of these numbers to practice the self-acupressure techniques in this book. But you might be interested in looking at meridian charts, in which case you can use the identification number given in this book.

Finally, each point has a **name**, which translation from Chinese to English is not always easy (some points bear more than one translation...). The name is related to the point's main benefit or characteristic. It is sometimes clear (like in "Sea of Energy", or "Facial Beauty"), but often times too obscure for the western mind ("Jumping Circle", "Elegant Mansion"). Not very useful, then, but so poetic!

In this book, we focus on the anatomical landmarks.
The meridian identification letters are:

B = Bladder
GB = Gall Bladder
H = Heart
K= Kidneys
LI = Large Intestine
Lu = Lungs
Lv = Liver
P = Pericardium
SI = Small Intestine
Sp = Spleen
St = Stomach
TW = Triple Warmer

How do I work the points?

There are several different techniques, including movement, rhythm and pressure, to work on the acupoints, which make for different acupressure styles. It goes from the softest (just lightly touching the point) to the hardest (deep firm penetration).

The techniques depend on the point location: points sitting on a strong ropy muscle call for firmness, whereas points sitting on fragile areas (e.g.: around the eyes) can take light touch only.

They also depend on the desired effect: pressing with an intermittent, fast beat is stimulating; a slower pressure creates a deeply relaxing effect on the body; tapping generates vibrations and "awakens' the whole meridian.

In this book, we'll use the following easy techniques:

Firm steady pressure is the most common technique. The thumbs are mainly used, but the others fingers, the palms, and the knuckles are often useful to apply stationary pressure.
There are two ways to apply pressure:
   - Hold the point without any movement for a few seconds to several minutes at a time.

- A series of short, firm pressures lasting a few seconds, about eight to twelve times.

Firm pressure with rotation: After applying steady, firm pressure directly on the acupoint, massage it with a slow rotating movement. Keep the circular movement small, so that you keep stimulating the right spot. Start with light pressure and gradually build up to a level before pain.

Rubbing uses brisk friction to stimulate the blood and lymph. It is appropriate for larger areas of the body, such as the back. Make a loose fist, and rub the skin lightly with your knuckles.

How do I apply pressure?

Always use the pulp of your finger tips, not the tip itself:

Yes:

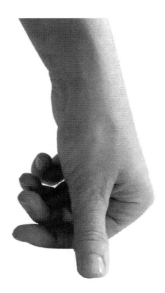

No:

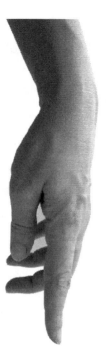

Depending on the point, you can use one or more fingers:

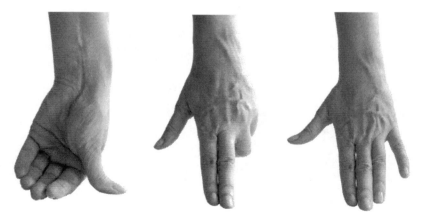

Whatever the technique, there are **3 steps to follow**:

1. Place your finger lightly on the point, as to make a gentle connection.
2. Begin building the pressure gently, at a 90 degree angle from the surface of the skin, and deepen it gradually.
3. Release the pressure slowly, but faster than the build-up.

A golden rule is to **use your body weight** instead of your muscle strength. That way, you do not tire your hands and arms. Whenever anatomically possible, **lean forward** into the point.

To spare your thumb, support it with the other fingers of the same hand, or use paired thumbs.

Tip: If your hand hurts, use tools such as a golf ball or a pencil eraser.

Finally, each acupoint feels differently when you press it. But always remember that **pain is not necessary**! The pressure should be firm enough so that it "hurts good" (in Chinese: "the exquisite pain"). Efficiency is NOT measured by the level of pain you experience. Some acupressure techniques use very light touch, yet they are extremely powerful.

If you feel extreme (or increasing) sensitivity or pain, gradually decrease the pressure until you find a balance between pain and pleasure. After working on the point for a few days, you will discover that the pain will diminish.

What else should I do?

Get prepared:

- Wear comfortable clothing
Tight pants, tops, collars, belts, or shoes can obstruct circulation. It is recommended to wear natural fibers that breathe, such as cotton, linen, silk or wool blends. Also, try to keep your fingernails trimmed fairly short to prevent any discomfort or injury to the skin.

- Don't fill your stomach

Digestion takes up to 60% of the body's energy. Wait until at least an hour after eating a light meal and even longer after eating a heavy meal. Avoid iced drinks (especially during the winter months), because extreme cold generally weakens your system and can counteract the benefits of acupressure.

- Avoid alcohol

Alcohol seriously disturbs the energy flow, as well as many vital organs.

Practice in a relaxing environment:

Greater benefits are achieved with deep relaxation. Whenever possible, create a comfortable, private environment. Choose a room where you will not be disturbed, and inform your entourage you need to be alone for 15mn.
You can burn essential oils, or light incense, play soft music, light candles, and even stay in the dark, whatever suits you.

Breathe deeply:

Concentrate on breathing slowly and deeply while you practice. Deep breathing helps to regulate your metabolism, enhancing the benefits of the exercises and massage. Long and deep breathing brings more oxygen in the body cells, and the organs function better. It helps your body heal itself, and induces relaxation.

When working on a sore or painful acupoint, focus your attention on the painful spot, inhale deeply, and imagine that you are breathing healing energy into the affected area. Do not use a rotation movement. Exhale slowly, letting the healing energy circulate throughout your body. Repeat for three full minutes. It will close the nervous system's pain gates and help the area heal. This breathing technique enhances the healing benefits of all the acupressure exercises in this book.

Practice regularly:

For optimal results, and to prevent recurrence, you should practice daily, even after you have obtained relief. If you cannot practice every day, try to treat yourself two or three times a week.

Close the session:

Following your routine, give yourself a few minutes to deeply relax on your back with your eyes closed. When you have only a couple of minutes at the end of the routine to relax, you can let yourself relax in a sitting position. First, rub the palms of your hands together briskly to create heat. Close your eyes and immediately place your hands lightly over your face as you breathe deeper than you normally breathe. After a minute, let your hands float into your lap and completely relax for a couple of minutes to discover the benefits.

Having a cup of hot herbal tea is a good idea after an acupressure session along with a period of deep relaxation.

Module 3:

Acupressure Points
for Weight Loss

Control your cravings

Boost your metabolism

Improve your digestion

Dissolve water retention

Boost your energy

Manage your stress

Acupressure for weight loss

Weight loss is a goal for many people and there are so many weight loss programs available. High protein diets and intensive cardio workouts, restricting the intake of carbs, one food-focused diets and strength building exercises... The choice of methods to try is so wide that it looks easy to succeed!

But it is *not* as easy. Sticking to an actual healthy routine is a change of lifestyle that needs a great deal of effort. Also, we have to be very careful about our diet as we need to supply our body with all the nutrients it needs to function properly.

How Can Acupressure Help?

According to the concepts of Traditional Chinese Medicine (TCM, of which acupressure is a branch), the reason for excess weight is an imbalance within different organ systems. For instance, the spleen focuses on the digestive functions, and disharmony within it can cause symptoms such as slow metabolism, fatigue and water retention.

As you read in Module 2 of this book, all the vital organs are regulated by an energy meridian, and acupressure (and acupuncture) is a way to access those systems through the points on the meridians.
Working on specific acupressure points regulates the flow of vital energy through the energy meridians. This energy flow balances your appetite, digestive system, metabolism and compulsive urges to eat.
That is why acupressure is very efficient to balance any such dysfunction. The objective is to harmonize the entire body system, including the physical (e.g.: digestive), emotional, nervous and endocrine spheres.

Acupressure therapy is also effective for healing your body's self-image and restoring your trust and awareness of its integrity. Acupressure is touch, and is self-care. Giving yourself acupressure sessions enables you to be more in touch with your body (literally!)

Finally, on an even higher level, acupressure can make you tune to the messages your body sends. With time it can develop a greater awareness and a deep, natural intuition about when and what to eat.

Of course, acupressure alone is not enough. You need a healthy diet and regular exercise, and you can add essential oils, herbs, supplements, breathing exercises and abdominal massages to your weight loss program.

How does the Program work?

The acupressure points and exercises described in this book fall in 4 categories:

- **Hunger Points**: to control compulsive eating and to relieve hunger.
- **Digestion Points**: to regulate the digestive process.
- **Endocrine Points**: to help the metabolism and prevent water retention.
- **Stress Points**: to reduce stress and calm the mind.

You will find a description of all the points, how to locate them and how to stimulate them. Start your program by getting familiar with those points and your unique body topography. Work on them one by one, anytime, especially if they are sore.

When you feel comfortable (it shouldn't take more than a week to explore the points and be confident), practice all the exercises described in the program.

Build your routine (series of exercises or points) depending on how you feel. By practicing it twice daily, you'll experience less stress, better appetite balance, and a greater sense of wellness.

As always, it is recommended that you consult your general physician before starting any new treatment.

... And don't forget to exercise! Even walking around the block is a good start. No excuses.

CONTROL YOUR CRAVINGS

The acupressure points described in this chapter regulate the digestive system and appetite. Their stimulation does not reduce or suppress appetite, it regulates it. In other words, it progressively shifts your body towards a *natural* level of hunger and a decrease in sugar cravings (and other appetite disorders).

Press the points for 60 seconds to 3 minutes. Try working these points as often as you can during the day.

Abbreviations and names are given for your reference if you would like to research more about the points.

RIB POINT:

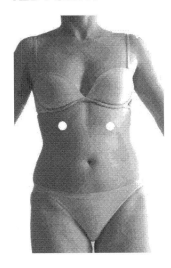

This point is located on the meridian that irrigates the spleen, so it regulates the gastrointestinal system.

It is known to relieve indigestion, ulcers, to balance acidity in the stomach, appetite imbalances, abdominal cramps, rib pain, and hiccups.

Names:
Spleen 16 (Sp16), Fu Ai, Abdominal Sorrow

Where:
Below the edge of the rib cage (at the junction of the 9th rib cartilage to the 8th rib), in line with your earlobe

How:
Curve your fingers, placing your fingertips in the indentation underneath the edge of the ribs. Press firmly in the indentations for one minute, and breathe slowly.

If you are standing up, press upward and lean your body forward to use your body weight for pressure.

EAR POINT:

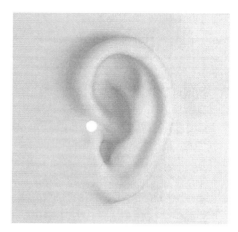

This appetite control point can help you avoid overeating. Begin your acupressure session stimulating these points (one on each ear). I suggest that you end your session by stimulating them again

Names:
Ear point #88, The Hunger Point

Where:
The point is situated just beneath your earlobe, where the skin of the ear is connected to the jaw.

How:
While looking in a mirror, place your fingers on your jaw, in front of your ears.
Open and close your mouth a few times until you feel your jaw bone moving underneath your fingers.
Put one finger where you feel the most movement of the jaw. Your finger should be right next to a little fleshy protrusion of the ear (not the ear lobe).
Grab this part of the ear with your thumb and index finger and press with steady pressure.

n.b.: The Stomach point is located nearby. Massage this area with your forefinger.

UPPER LIP POINT:

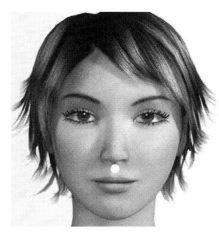

Names:
Governing Vessel 26, GV26, Shui Gou, Water Trough

Where:
Between the upper lip and the nose. To be exact it is one third of the way from the nose.

How:
Place your thumb under your upper lip, and your index finger on the outside. Press or manipulate this area with a moderate pressure for 60 seconds to few minutes.

BOOST YOUR METABOLISM

The thyroid gland, located at the base of the throat, works on a physiological level to balance your metabolism rate.

NECK POINTS:

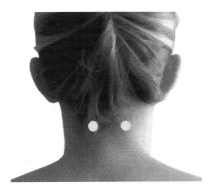

The most healing thyroid points are localized near your thyroid gland and are called the *Windows to the Sky*. These points are stimulated effectively in the following exercise called the Butterfly Neck Press. For best results, you need to do this exercise 3 to 5 times daily for a few months.

How:
Interlace your fingers behind your neck.

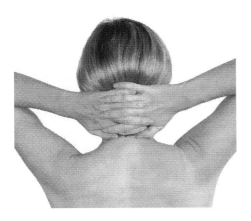

While inhaling deeply, lean your head back and bring your elbows out stretching the chest area open. Hold for 3 counts.
On the exhalation, slowly drop your head forward, bringing the elbows close together, touching if possible. Hold for another 3 counts.

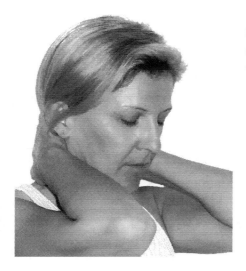

Repeat 4 more times, inhaling up and exhaling down to release any tension in your neck.

Then continue with the use of the Collarbone Points.

COLLARBONE POINTS:

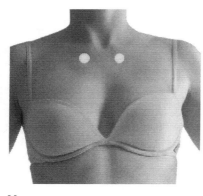

Names:
Kidneys 27, K27, Yu Fu, Elegant Mansion.

Where:
In the hollow below the collarbone next to the breastbone. If you press firmly, these points can be sore.

How:
Use the middle finger of both hands, or the thumb and middle finger of one hand.

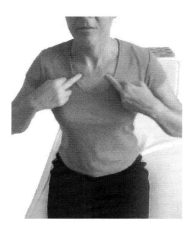

The pressure should be very light. Touch is enough (just place the finger pulp, and do not press). These acupoints are sensitive and reactive. You can feel the pulse just below the skin.

Close your eyes, take long, slow deep breaths as you slowly let your head turn from side to side.

Feel your entire neck region relax as you continue to breathe deeply, while holding these points.

Gently let your head tilt upward as you inhale and downward as you exhale, while you use your mind to visualize more blood flowing through your thyroid gland at the base of your throat. Hold the points for 30 seconds minimum, 1 minute if possible.

With your hands in your lap, take another minute or two to let yourself completely relax.

Be sure to practice the Butterfly Neck Press breathing exercise followed by holding the K 27 acupressure points 3 to 5 times daily for at least 3 months.
Once you begin to achieve results and your thyroid balances, you will still need to do these practices, but not as many times per day, for maintenance and prevention.

THUMB POINT:

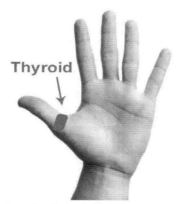

Thyroid

On the hands, the area related to the thyroid is located at the base of the thumb, on the inner side (palm side), just above the palm cushion. Massaging it stimulates the thyroid and increases the metabolism. Massage this area with a strong intention to activate the thyroid.

Massage this area for around three minutes, before moving slightly farther up the fleshy pad, toward the wrist, and continue massaging to stimulate the pancreas. This will help regulate insulin production and keep your blood-sugar levels steady. Spikes in blood sugar can cause hunger pangs and an increase in appetite for sweet, sugar-laden foods.

IMPROVE YOUR DIGESTION

By stimulating acupressure points you work on your organs: as seen in the first part of this book, each energy meridian (on which the points are located) is associated to a physical vital organ. By working on the Spleen, Stomach and Large Intestine meridians, acupressure can improve the digestive process.

INNER LEG POINT:

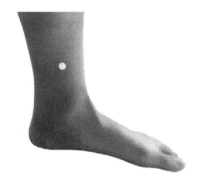

This is one of the most commonly used points and one of the most versatile. Because the point crosses the Spleen, Kidney and Liver meridians, it can treat many conditions associated with all three organs. It's an important point in the treatment of any digestive, gynaecological and emotional condition. It has a strengthening effect on the digestive system.

Names:
Spleen 6, Sp6, San Yin Jiao, Three Yin Intersection.

Where:
This point is located on the inner side of the leg, above the ankle bone. From the center of the ankle bone, slide up four finger widths. The point is just off the bone, toward the back of the leg.

How:

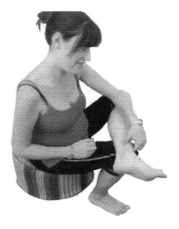

When you find it, press with your thumb or knuckle. Increase pressure until you are pressing quite firmly, hold about a minute, and gradually release.

Caution: Do not press this point if you are pregnant.

OUTER LEG POINT:

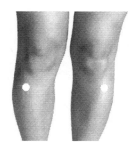

This point is the best point to nourish the chi and blood, boost digestion and promote general wellness.

Names:
Stomach 36, St36, Zusanli, Three Miles

Where:
St 36 is located four finger widths below the lower border of the kneecap and one finger width off the shin bone to the outside.

This point is one of the most difficult to locate. You've found the point correctly if you feel the muscle move under your fingers when you flex your foot up and down.

How:
Because it is located in a thick muscular area, it requires strong pressure.

There are 2 positions to work this point:

- Sit, legs bent, feet flat on the floor. Press with your thumbs, or rub the points with your knuckles or roll a small ball on each point. Press as hard as you can.

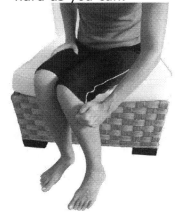

- Sit, legs stretched on the floor. Lean your body forward to apply a vertical pressure. This technique is more relaxing, and more efficient.

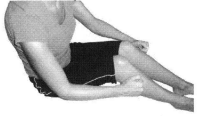

Using moderate to firm pressure, hold for about one minute.
Stimulate both points in the morning, and after lunch

ELBOW POINT:

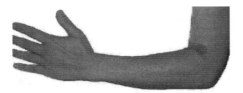

If you are in a situation where massaging your ears or face is not appropriate, you can press this point more discreetly. This point helps to regulate intestinal activity and clear excess heat and moisture from the body

Names:
Large Intestine 11, LI11, Qu Chi, Crooked Pond

Where:
The outer elbow point is located on the outer end of the elbow crease. Hold your arm in front of your chest, as if holding a cup in your hand. The point is at the outside end of the crease on your arm at the elbow joint. Another way to find it is to note the length of your thumb from the tip to the first joint, then move this distance up from the outside tip of the elbow bone toward the crease lines at the elbow joint.

How:
Bend your arms and press the outer end of the crease into your elbow.

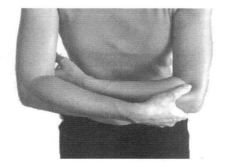

Use firm pressure with your right thumb. Press for about 60 seconds to few minutes.
Then switch arms.

DISSOLVE WATER RETENTION

There are five pressure points on the body that are believed to help with water retention. Working on these points can help you get better quicker.

You do not have to use all of these points. Using just one or two of them whenever you have a free hand can be effective.

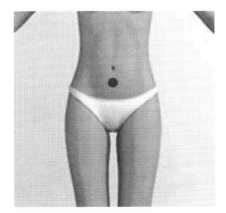 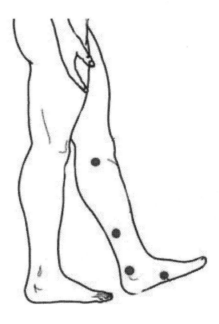

TUMMY POINT:

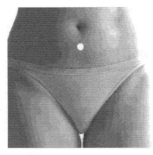

Relieves water retention, chronic diarrhoea, constipation, and gas.

Names:
Conception Vessel 6 (CV6), Sea of Energy, Hara

Where:
Two finger widths directly below the belly button.

How:
You can place your three middle fingers of either hand, on the point area, and press down an inch or two until you reach a firm spot.

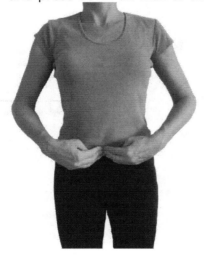

Or, you can use a more relaxed hold and place the palm of one hand gently on your belly, below your belly button, right over the point. You can use one hand, or both, with one hand over the other.

Remember to relax your hands and arms and shoulders. You can hold this while standing (evenly on both feet), sitting (with both feet flat on the ground, back straight), or lying down.

Hold for one or two minutes, while taking slow deep breaths.

UPPER INNER LEG POINT:

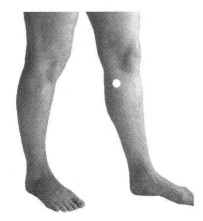

This point is known to relieve water retention but also knee problems, swelling, leg tension, varicose veins, oedema and cramps.

Names:
Spleen 9, Sp9, Shady Side of the Mountain, Yin Ling Quan.

Where:
On the inside of the leg in the depression right below a rounded prominence in the top of the leg bone (tibia).

How:
Place your left thumb on the right leg point and press in the depression, slightly upwards.
Remember to relax your shoulders. Hold for one or two minutes, while taking slow deep breaths.
Switch sides: place your right thumb on the left leg point, press in the depression, slightly upwards, relax your shoulders, old for one or two minutes, while taking slow deep breaths.

LOWER INNER LEG POINT:

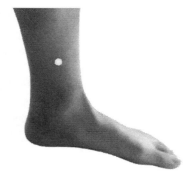

This point is very versatile. It sits where the Spleen, Kidney and Liver meridians intersect and is a very powerful point. It can treat many conditions associated with all three organs. If you have digestive, gynaecological or emotional conditions, just find the point and massage it. It may be tender, but do this for two minutes. The tenderness should subside and so should the symptoms.

Names:

Spleen 6, Sp6, San Yin Jiao, Three Yin Intersection.

Where:

This point is located on the inner side of the leg (on the back inner border of the shinbone), four finger widths above the inner anklebone.

How:

Sit down and place your left ankle on your right knee. Place your right hand fingers (except the thumb) on the area above the ankle. That will help you locate the point.

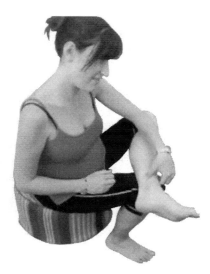

Press with your thumb or knuckle. Increase pressure until you are pressing quite firmly, hold about a minute, and gradually release. Switch legs and work on the right leg point.

Caution: Do not press this point if you are pregnant.

LOWER INNER LEG POINT:

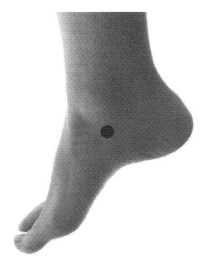

This point is another very versatile acupressure point. I include it in this Weight Loss Program because it relieves water retention and oedema in the legs, especially swollen ankles. In addition it relieves sore throat, swollen, dry, loss of voice, difficulty swallowing, a range of menstrual issues (amenorrhea, dysmenorrhoea, infertility from cold in the uterus, leucorrhoea), genital issues (swelling, itching, seminal emission), constipation,   insomnia and disturbed sleep with nightmares, and a range of anxiety disorders!

Names:
Kidney 6, K6, Zhao Hai, Shining Sea or Illuminated Sea.

Where:
This point is located one thumb width below the inside of the anklebone.

How:
Proceed as for acupressure point Spleen 6: sit down and place your left ankle on your right knee. Place your right thumb in the depression right below the ankle bone.
Press with your thumb or knuckle. Increase pressure until you are pressing quite firmly, hold about a minute, and gradually release.
Switch legs and work on the right leg point.

FOOT POINT:

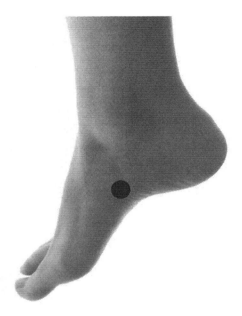

Relieves oedema, especially swollen feet.

Names:
Kidney 2, K2, Ran Gu, Blazing Valley.

Where:
This point is located on the middle of the arch of the foot, midway between the outer tip of the big toe and the back of the heel.

How:
Sit down and place your left ankle on your right knee. Place your right thumb in the depression of the arch. With your thumb perpendicular to the arch, apply firm pressure in the direction of the inner center of the foot. Press with your thumb or knuckle. Increase pressure until you are pressing quite firmly, hold about a minute, and gradually release.
Switch legs and work on the right foot point.

BOOST YOUR ENERGY

When our metabolism is high, we digest more efficiently, so when we eat the same amount of food, we don't feel hungry shortly after.

An efficient way to stimulate your metabolism is to increase your general energy level.

For a sugar-free energy boost, work on the following points, commonly used to treat weakness, fatigue and exhaustion. The points described below are each efficient for a specific kind of fatigue. Choose the one(s) that fit your condition and work on it/them anytime, for a few minutes each time.

You will also find exercises at the end of the chapter to use several points in one routine.

PRIMAL ENERGY:

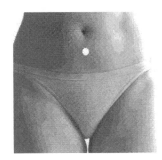

This point alone can enable you to lose weight by stimulating your body's energy to eliminate properly. It also increases the strength and function of your intestines.

Names:
Conception Vessel 6 (CV6), Qi Hai, Sea of Energy, Hara

Where:
Two finger widths directly below the belly button.

How:

You can place your three middle fingers of either hand, on the point area, and press down an inch or two until you reach a firm spot.

Or, you can use a more relaxed hold and place the palm of one hand gently on your belly, below your belly button, right over the point. You can use one hand, or both, with one hand over the other.

Remember to relax your hands and arms and shoulders. You can hold this while standing (evenly on both feet), sitting (with both feet flat on the ground, back straight), or lying down.

Hold for one or two minutes, while taking slow deep breaths.

PHYSICAL STAMINA AND ENDURANCE:

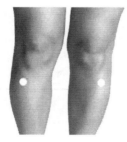

This point is commonly used for stress and fatigue as well as for gastrointestinal discomfort.

Names:
Stomach 36, St36, Zu San Li, Three Miles

Where:
St 36 is located four finger widths below the lower border of the kneecap and one finger width off the shin bone to the outside.

This point is one of the most difficult to locate. You've found the point correctly if you feel the muscle move under your fingers when you flex your foot up and down.

How:
This point being in a thick muscular area, it requires strong pressure.
There are 2 positions to work this point:

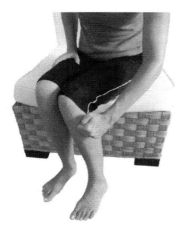

Sit, legs bent, feet flat on the floor. Press with your thumbs, or rub the points with your knuckles or roll a small ball on each point. Press as hard as you can.

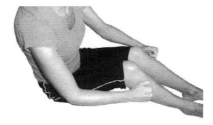

Sit, legs stretched on the floor. Lean your body forward to apply a vertical pressure. This technique is more relaxing, and more efficient.

Using moderate to firm pressure, hold for about one minute.
Stimulate this point in the morning, and after lunch

GENERAL TIREDNESS:

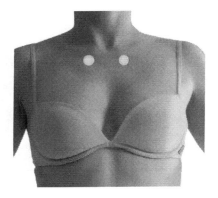

The 27th and last point on the Kidney meridians is the neurological centre of the acupuncture circuit. This main switchboard is an important organizer of energy flow throughout the body.

The K-27s are commonly used for the following conditions:
- Low energy
- Tired all the time
- Low immunity
- Always sick
- Jet lag

Names:
Elegant Mansion, Kidneys 27

Where:
They are located between the clavicle and the first rib up against the breastbone. In the hollow below the collarbone next to the breastbone.
If you press firmly, these points can be sore.

How:

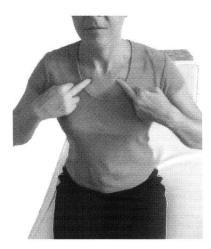

Use the right hand to stimulate the left K-27 and the left hand to stimulate the right K-27 for easier access and leverage, while the opposite hand is placed over the navel. It is important to always ground at the navel.

Position the middle finger of both hands on the two points at the same time, or use the thumb and middle finger of one hand.

The pressure should be very light. Touching is enough (just place the fleshy part of the finger tip, and do not press).

These acupoints are sensitive and reactive. You can feel the pulse just below the skin. Close your eyes, and hold the points for 30 seconds minimum, 1 minute if possible.

EXHAUSTION, CHRONIC FATIGUE:

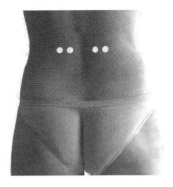

Names:
Bladder 23 and Bladder 47

Where:
In the lower back, at waist level, between the second and third lumbar vertebrae, 2 to 4 finger widths away from the spine.

B23 : 2 finger widths away from the spine.
B47 : 4 finger widths away from the spine.

How:
There are 2 ways to work on these points:

Stand up or sit down:
Place your hands on your waist, thumbs on the back. Press the points with your thumbs.
Or rub the points with the back of your hands.

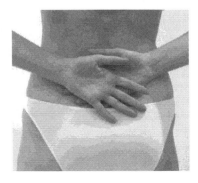

Lie down on your back: place 2 small balls on the floor, at the level of B23 and B47. Let the weight of your body do the pressure work.

For a softer stimulation, place your hands under your waist, palms on the floor, knuckles up on B23 and B47.

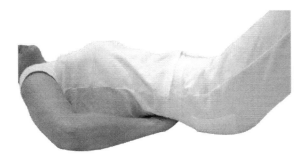

Caution: Do not press on disintegrating discs or fractured or broken bones, If you have a weak back, a few minutes of stationary, light touching instead of pressure can be very healing. See your doctor first if you have any questions or need medical advice.

AGE-RELATED FATIGUE & LOW ENERGY:

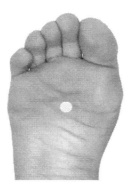

The kidney meridian, also known as "The Minister of Power" is the most important reservoir of energy in the body. Our original qi (transmitted by our parents during conception and that decreases with time) is stored in the kidney. This energy is released from the kidney during any time of increased stress. This leaves the kidneys very low on energy at the end of the day...

K1 is the first point on that meridian and the energy bubbles its way up from there.

It also connects us deeply with the Earth-energy (since we stand up). We might imagine sending roots down through the soles of our feet, like a tree, all the way to the centre of the Earth. As we connect in this way deeply with the Earth, we feel both stable and energized.

Names:
Kidney 1, K1, Yong Quan, Bubbling Spring

Where:
On the centre of the sole of the foot, at the base of the ball of the foot, between the two pads.

How:
Sit down on the floor, and
Use your thumb to gradually press on K1. The circular motion technique can also be used.

If you sit on a chair, comfortably rest the ankle of your left leg over the knee or thigh of the right leg. Then, cradle your left foot in your right hand, while using your right thumb or knuckles to massage - with moderate to deep pressure.

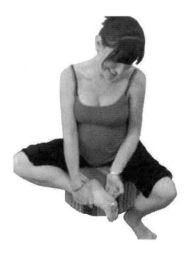

Continue for 2-3 minutes, and then switch sides.

EXERCISE #1: General fatigue

Lie down on your back, with your knees bent and your feet flat on the floor. This daily routine can be done sitting, although it is less effective.

1. Firmly press CV6 (abdomen):

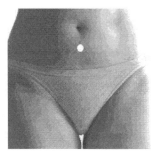

Place all your fingertips of both hands between the pubic bone and the belly button. Take long deep breaths as you gradually press 1 or 2 inches deep inside the abdomen, and as you apply firm pressure for 1mn.

Caution: Press this point LIGHTLY if you have had a recent abdominal operation, or if you have serious, life-threatening illness (heart disease, cancer, high blood pressure).

2. Lightly press Sp9 and Sp6 (inner leg):

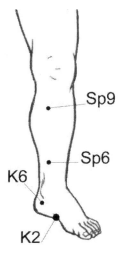

With your legs bent and your feet flat on the floor, place your right foot comfortably on your left thigh. Use your right thumb to gently press the right Sp9 point. Use your left thumb to press Sp6. Close your eyes, and breathe deeply for 1mn. Hold the points lightly for another 2 long breaths. Then switch legs.

3. Press K2 and K6 (foot):

Place your foot as in Step 2. Use your right fingertips to press the right K6. Place your left thumb on the right K2. Hold these points for 1mn. Then switch legs. Breathe deeply.

EXERCISE #2: Rejuvenate

Lie down on your back, knees bent, feet flat on the floor.

1. Place the knuckles of your lose fist on the B47 points in your back (the right fist if the right side of your back is tenser than the left side, the left fist if the left side of your back is tenser).

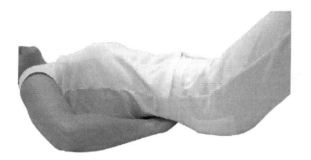 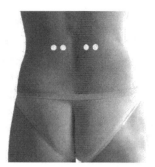

2. With the other hand, **hold B10, K27, CV12 and CV6** in this order for 1mn each. For the double points, hold only the one located on the opposite side of the fist under your back:

B10:   K27:

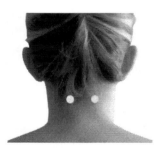   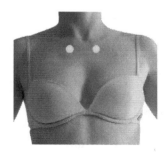

CV12:

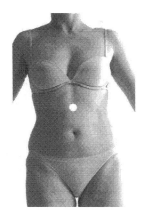

CV6:

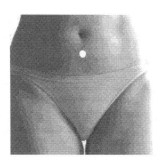

3. Press both Sp13 (pelvic area):

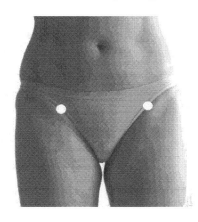

Place all the fingers of both hands on Sp13, located in the middle of the crease where the leg joins the trunk of the body:

4. Firmly press St36 (below the knee):

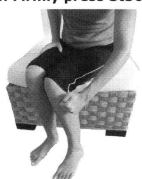

Keep your legs bent, feet flat on the floor, and sit down. Press your thumbs into St36, four finger widths below the kneecap toward the outside of the shinbone:

EXERCISE #3: Regulate your energy

1. Lie down on your back, knees bent, feet flat on the floor. Place the middle finger of your left hand on the left B10 point in the back of your neck.

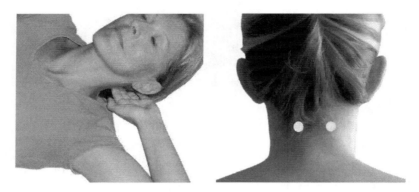

2. With the right hand, **hold St3, and then Sp13** for 1mn each. Hold only the right acupoint.

St3:   Sp13:

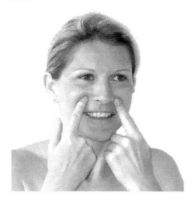   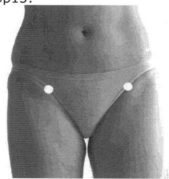

3. Place your right foot on your left knee
Hold at the same time K3 (inner ankle) with your thumb, **and B60 (outer ankle)** with your middle finger for 1mn.

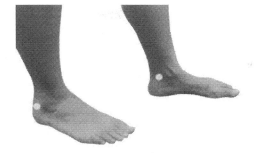

4. With your right hand, hold the toes of your right foot, then left foot.

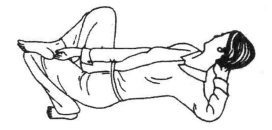

MANAGE YOUR STRESS

Being under stress worsens eating disorders. The points and exercises in this chapter reduce stress and are easy to practice. In less than a half-hour, practicing once or twice a day, you can greatly lower your anxiety, emotional stress and swings, and indirectly transform your metabolism, appetite, and tame your eating disorders.

TOP OF THE FOOT POINT:

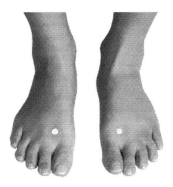

Liver 3 (Lv 3) prevents Chi stagnation in the body and is the most important point for combating stress. It is also very efficient for detox and decongestion.

Names: Liver 3, Lv 3, Tai Chong, Great Surge.

Where:
Lv 3 is situated on top of your foot in the webbing between your big toe and second toe.

How:
Sit down on a chair or sofa. Place you feet on the floor or cross your legs.

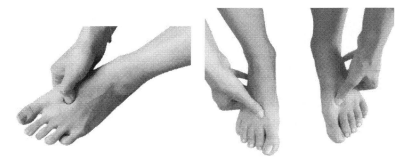

Start at the web margin of skin between the two toes, and slide your index finger up between the bones until you feel a depression about 1/2 inch up.

Using your thumb or forefinger, press between the bones (in the direction of the root of the second toe). Start with light pressure, as this point can be sensitive, and increase as much as you can until you are using moderate to firm pressure. Press for about 1 minute.

Alternative: Rub it with your heel.

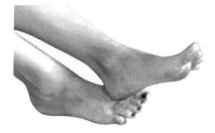

Sit down on a chair or sofa and place your feet flat on the floor.
Lift your right foot, and place its heel on your left Lv3. Rub the area for up to 1 minute.
Then switch sides.

MENTAL STRESS:

Appetite can be disturbed in case of mental stress. To calm your mental stress, try this gentle acupressure exercise. It is as efficient as a short meditation. Practice before and during eating, to avoid relieving stress with food, and to promote good digestion.

A Mini-meditation with acupoints

This exercise is for those who find it difficult to meditate, and/or have little time to do it.
Meditation is a powerful source of health and well-being. Even if you do not have enough free time to practice regularly and fully, a few moments of deep breathing while working on specific acupressure points are enough to help you calm down and center.

It takes a few minutes only, and can be practiced anywhere: sitting at your desk, in a taxi, lying on a bed or on a sofa.

It is easy to do, and it stimulates two important acupoints/chakras: the Third Eye (between the eyebrows), and the Hara (below the navel).

1. Standing up or comfortably seated, close your eyes. Relax your shoulders.

2. Gently put the cushion of your middle finger on the Third Eye (between the eyebrows), and the palm of your other hand on the Hara (between the navel and the pubic bone).

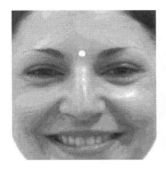 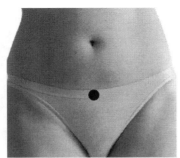

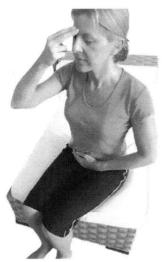

3. Take 5 long... deep.... Breaths...

4. Slowly open your eyes and smile!

EMOTIONAL STRESS:

Cravings are often triggered by emotional stress. To balance your emotions, stimulate the following point:

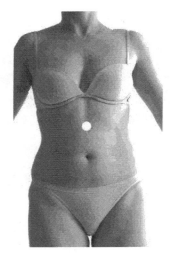

Names:
Conception Vessel 12, CV12, Center of Power.

Where:
This point is located on the Solar Plexus chakra, hence is name.
More precisely, it is sitting in the centre of the abdomen, on the midline between the base of the breastbone and the belly button.

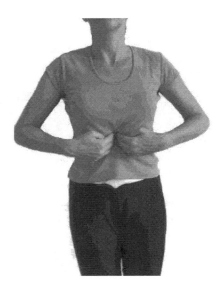

How:
Standing up, sitting down, or ling on your back, place all the fingertips of both hands along the midline below the breastbone.

Press *gradually*, at an upward angle toward the center of your back. You can lean your body forward. Breathe deeply as you hold for one minute.

Caution: In general, it is recommended to work this point for not more than 2 minutes, and not right after a meal.
Do not press firmly on this point or rub it briskly or tap it if you have a serious illness.

MOOD SWINGS:

Key Acupressure points:

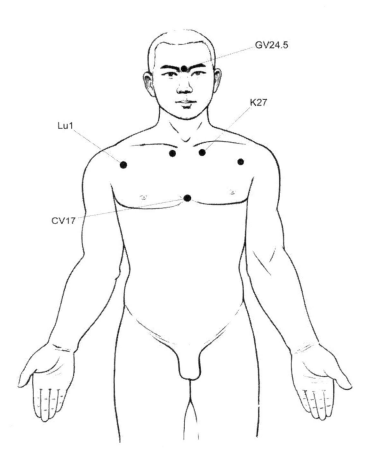

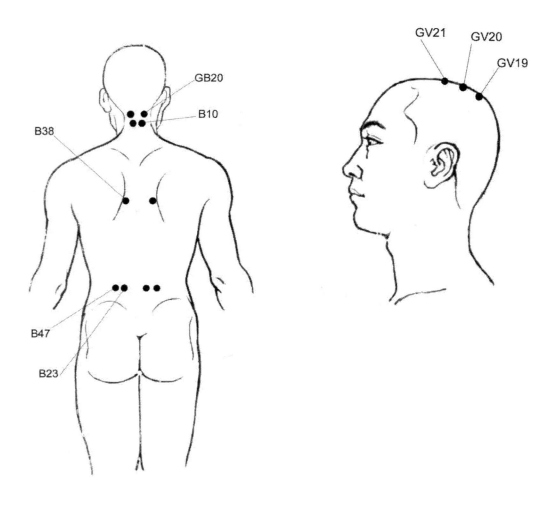

EXERCISE:

Concentrate on breathing slowly and deeply throughout all of the steps. Deep breathing increases circulation to every part of your body, washes away tension, relieves depression, and infuses your body with vitality.

Lie down on your back:

1. Press B38 (upper back):

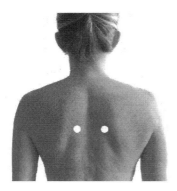

Lie down on your back, and place 2 golf or tennis table balls on the floor underneath your upper back between your shoulder blades. If the pressure hurts, cover the balls with a thick towel. Close your eyes, and breathe for 2mn.

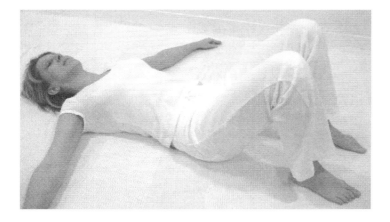

2. Firmly press B10 and GB20 (neck):

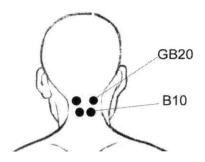

Use your fingertips to firmly press B10 on both sides of the ropy muscles on your neck for 1mn. Then use your thumbs to gradually press up underneath the skull into GB20, as you slowly tilt your head back and breathe deeply for another minute.

3. Stimulate GV19, GV20 and GV21 (top of the head):

Place your fingertips on the centre on the top of your head, and then briskly rub with all your fingertips to stimulate these 3 antidepressant points for 1mn.

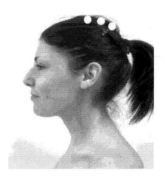

4. Firmly press K27 and Lu1 (upper chest):

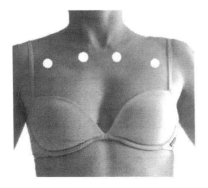

Use your fingertips on both sides of your chest to firmly press K27 and then Lu1 for 1mn each.

Slowly sit up and continue.

5. Rub B23 and B47 (lower back):
Make fists and place your knuckles against your lower back, 2 inches apart on either side of the spine. Briskly rub your back up and down for 1mn to create heat.

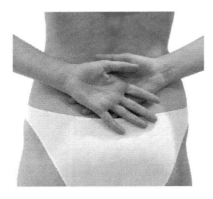 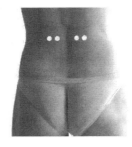

6. Rub St36 (lower leg):

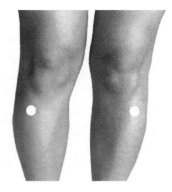

Place your left fist on St36 of your left leg and briskly rub it for 1mn. Then do the same on the other leg.

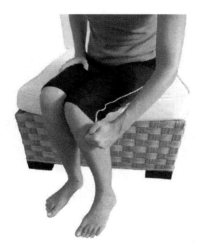

7. Third Eye visualization:

Sitting with your spine straight, eyes closed, chin tilted down slightly, bring your palms together and use your middle and index fingertips to lightly touch the Third Eye point.

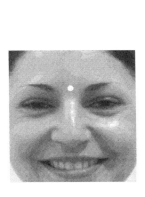
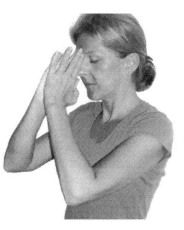

Take long, slow, deep breaths as you visualize yourself going to a place that makes you feel calm, restful, and safe – a place where you can trust yourself to follow whatever step you need to take to reach fulfillment in your life.

Use all of the fingertips of one hand to gently press the centre of your breastbone as you take several more long, slow, deep breaths to enhance the benefits.

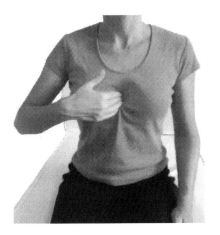
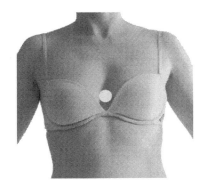

ANXIETY:

Key Acupressure points:

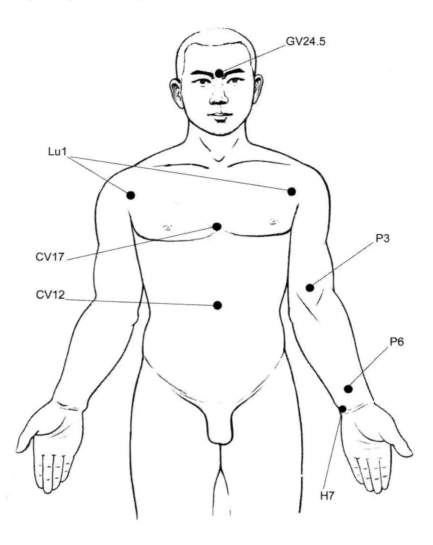

EXERCISE:

1. Breathe

Stand with your feet comfortably apart and your arms at your sides. Inhale, raising your arms, palms up, out to the sides and then up above your head.

Interlock your fingers, with your palms facing each other. Turn your palms inside out so that your palms face the sky. Inhale, and gently stretch farther upward, with your head tilted back.
Exhale, lowering your chin to your chest and letting your arms float back down to your sides.
Repeat 5 times.

2. Press CV12 (stomach):

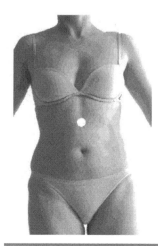

Place the fingertips of both hands between your belly button and the base of your breastbone. Gradually apply firm pressure in and upward, leaning your upper body forward, to press deeply into the pit of your stomach, as you breathe deeply for 1mn.

3. Press B48 and GB30 (buttocks):

Place your thumbs on the muscles of your buttocks to press B48 just below your lower back.

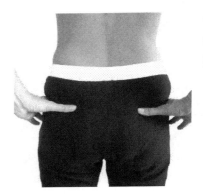

Take several long, slow, deep breaths as you firmly press inward (toward the centre of your pelvis) for 1mn.

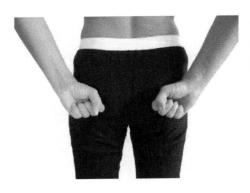

Then make fists and slide them one inch down and one inch outward to press GB30 for another minute.

4. Press Lu1 (upper outer chest):

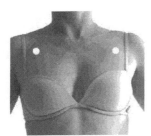

Place your thumbs on the upper, outer portion of your chest, feeling for tension there. Make firm contact with the muscles located 4 finger widths up and 1 finger width inward from your armpit. Close your eyes and concentrate on breathing deeply as you hold those chest points for 1mn.

5. Hold P3, press P6 and H7 (inner arm):

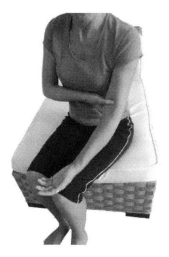

Hold P3 with your thumb:

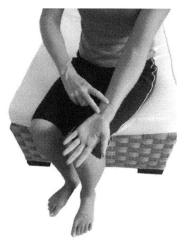

Press P6 and H7 with your forefinger and middle finger for 30 to 60 seconds each:

Then switch sides. If you continue to breathe slowly through your nose, you will find that your body is releasing its stress and nervous tension.

6. Hold GV24.5 with CV17 (face, sternum):

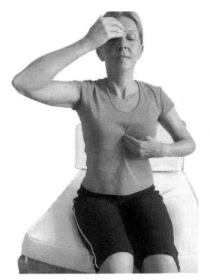

Gently place your right middle fingertip in between your eyebrows on GV24.5 in the slight indentation just above the bridge of the nose. Use the fingertips of your left hand to hold CV17 in the indentations in the centre of your breastbone. Close your eyes and breathe deeply into these points for at least 1mn.

Module 4:

DIY Acupressure Daily Routine for Weight Loss

Apply steady, penetrating finger pressure to each of the following points for 3 minutes.

1. Begin with the **Hunger ear point**. This appetite control point can help you avoid overeating. Begin your acupressure session stimulating this point. We suggest that you end your session by stimulating this point again.

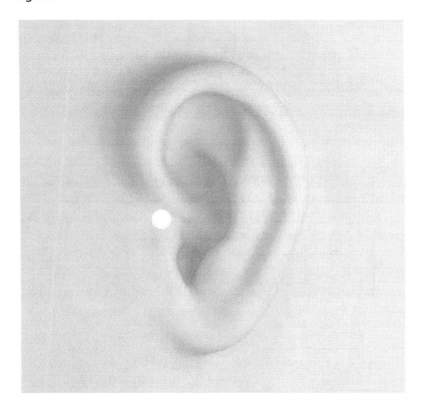

Locate the little fleshy protrusion of the ear (not the ear lobe). Grab this part of the ear with your thumb and index finger and press with steady pressure.

2. Spleen 6 (Sp 6) has a strengthening effect on the digestive system. This point is located on the interior side of your leg, above the ankle bone.

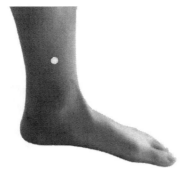

From the centre of the ankle bone, slide up four finger widths. The point is just off the bone, toward the back of the leg. When you find it, apply pressure with your thumb or knuckle. Increase pressure until you are pressing quite firmly, hold about a minute, and gradually release.

3. Stomach 36 (St 36) is the best point to nourish the Chi and blood. It has a beneficial effect on the digestive system.

St 36 is located four finger widths below the lower border of the kneecap and one finger width off the shin bone to the outside.

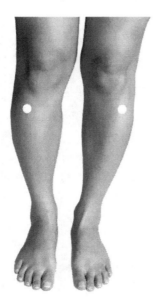

Flex your foot up and down. Feel the muscle move under your fingers. That's where the point is. Using moderate to firm pressure, hold for about one minute.

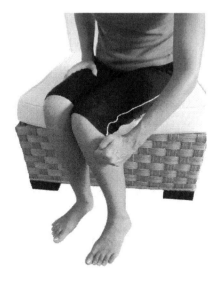 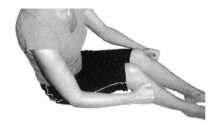

4. Spleen 9 (Sp 9) This point is close to St 36. After pressing St 36, slide your finger across the shinbone until you are just off the shinbone on the inside side of the leg. Now slide your finger upwards along the shinbone towards the knee about an inch, until you fall into a natural depression. Sp 9 is in this depression, right below a rounded prominence in the top of the leg bone (tibia). This point is involved with the metabolism of water in your body.

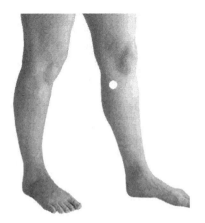 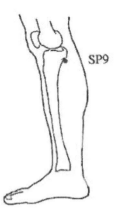

5. Stomach 40 (St 40) is an important point for clearing excess damp and phlegm. It is useful for eliminating excess weight.

St 40 is located midway between the ankle bone and the knee joint on the outside of the leg, three finger widths from the noticeable edge of the leg bone (fibula).

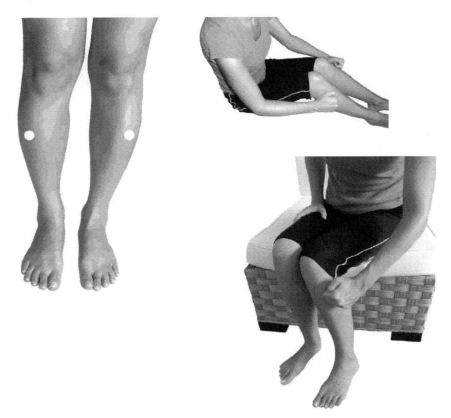

6. Large Intestine 11 (Li 11) is useful for clearing excess heat and damp from the body and to regulate the intestines activity.

Li 11 is located at the outer end of your elbow crease on the thumb side. Hold your arm in front of your chest, as if holding a cup in your hand. The point is at the outside end of the crease on your arm at the elbow joint.

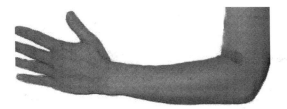

Another way to find it is to note the length of your thumb from the tip to the first joint, then move this distance up from the outside tip of the elbow bone toward the crease lines at the elbow joint. Hold your left hand close to your chest and use firm pressure with your right thumb; press for about a minute, then switch arms.

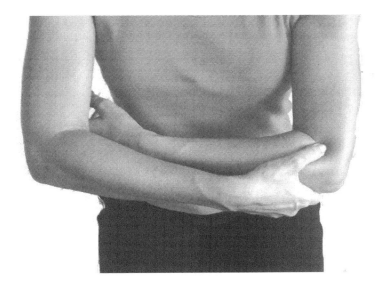

7. Liver 3 (Lv 3) prevents Chi stagnation in the body and is the most important point for fighting stress.

Lv 3 is situated on top of your foot in the webbing between your big toe and second toe.

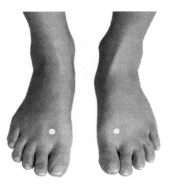

Start at the web margin of skin between the two toes, and slide your index finger up between the bones until you feel a depression about 1/2 inch up. Using your index finger, press between the bones (in the direction of the root of the second toe). Start with light pressure, as this point can be sensitive, and increase as much as you can until you are using moderate to firm pressure. Press for about 1 minute.

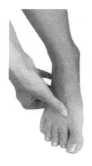
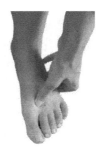
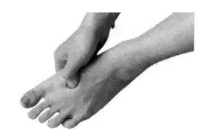

8. End your Acupressure session by stimulating again the appetite control point on both ears.

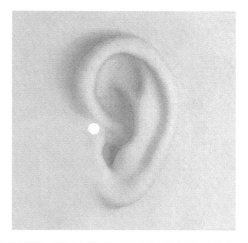

Module 5:

Essential Oils for
Natural Weight Loss

Using traditional Chinese medicine (TCM) and Acupressure for weight loss is a time-tested method as it addresses both the psychological and physiological aspects of reducing body weight.

There are other natural methods that can be used at the same time, thus increasing your chances of success.

You can harness the safe, natural fat-fighting properties of plants and fruit by supplementing your diet and fitness regimen with essential oils. Essential oils are a terrific and natural way to reduce appetite and calm emotions as they relate to food and stress, and actually dissolve fat.

You can also burn them while practicing your acupressure exercises. That is why I am adding a few recipes as a supplement to your DIY Acupressure Program.

Safety Precautions:

- Only use therapeutic grade essential oils when wanting healing results! Because they are approved as a Food Additive (FA) by the FDA, food grade oils are readily available on the market.
- Do not ingest oils that are not marked GRAS (Generally Regarded As Safe) or are not labeled for supplement use.
- Before applying, ingesting or inhaling any essential oil, make sure to read the instructions and precautions on every bottle.

Fenugreek Seeds Oil

Increases metabolism. Reduces appetite.

Fenugreek seed essential oil may have a positive role in supporting weight loss as both a metabolic enhancer and an appetite suppressant.
Increased metabolic output burns more energy and can accelerate fat loss. Fenugreek has the added benefit with regard to fat reduction in that it helps "break up" fat deposits in the bloodstream to be used as energy. Using energy sources the body already has stored can reduce the cravings for food.

Fenugreek Oil Weight Loss Recipe:
10 drops Fenugreek Oil
10 drops Cinnamon Oil
10 drops Bergamot Oil
10 drops Ginger Oil

Mix well and massage to the desired area.

Grapefruit Essential Oil

Increases metabolism.

Grapefruit has long been known for its numerous health benefits.
It is also one of the top essential oils for weight loss due mainly to the
large amounts of d-Limonene it contains.

D-Limonene is found in citrus peels and has a number of antioxidant and
anti-inflammatory uses alongside its natural weight management
properties. In a recent study, d-Limonene was given to rats for 45 days,
resulting in vast improvement in metabolic enzyme levels. Other animal
studies show that it reduces body weight and food intake, and can even
help lower cholesterol.

Grapefruit Oil Weight Loss Recipe:
Adding a few drops to a pint of water will make an invigorating and
refreshing drink that will do wonders for your weight.

Peppermint Essential Oil

Reduces cravings.

Peppermint essential oil can be a real help in reducing appetite – great if you are prone to cravings. It is also packed with nutrients, including vitamin C, omega-3 fatty acids, and minerals including potassium, iron and magnesium, meaning that it can help nourish the body while promoting weight loss.

This is great news when you consider that a 2008 study conducted by the Wheeling Jesuit University showed that when inhaling peppermint oil every two hours, participants experienced less hunger and fewer cravings than those who didn't use the oil.

It also works as a digestive aid which can soothe stomach upset while promoting a feeling of well-being.

Peppermint Oil Weight Loss Recipes:
A couple of drops in a glass of water after food will help digestion and stop you going back for a second helping.

Try adding a couple of drops to a warm bath every morning for a refreshing and appetite suppressing start to the day.

Bergamot Essential Oil

Reduces cholesterol levels. Increases metabolism.

Bergamot essential oil is extracted from the peel of Italian citrus fruits. Like peppermint oil, bergamot can help stimulate the endocrine system, creating a relaxed feeling of well-being. This is perfect for those who eat when stressed, or are prone to comfort eating.

It also contains an abundance of polyphenols (also found in green tea), which have been shown to increase metabolism and fat oxidation in studies.

Bergamot has also been shown to inhibit an enzyme (HMG-CoA), which reduces the bad LDL cholesterol in the blood. A 2009 study in the Journal on Natural Products compared bergamot to statins in its ability to lower cholesterol, reducing LDL levels from 20% – 59% (Statin 18% to 55%), while raising HDL levels from 7% to 83% (Statin 5% – 15%).

Bergamot Oil Weight Loss Recipe:
You can choose to either inhale peppermint oil before a meal or drink a few drops in a glass of water or tea right before each meal.

Lemon Essential Oil

Improves digestion. Boosts metabolism.

Like grapefruit and bergamot, lemon essential oil is absolutely packed with vitamins and minerals, especially Vitamin C. Lemon is most famously known for its cleaning abilities, and can be used to clean the hair and scalp as well as the digestive system and kidneys.

Like grapefruit, it also contains a large amount of d-Limonene, known for its metabolism boosting properties.

Lemon Oil Weight Loss Recipe:
Adding a couple of drops to a pint of water will create a refreshing, cleansing drink, which is perfect for hot summer days.
Since lemon essential oil is carminative, you can also use the drink to treat a number of stomach problems such as cramps, indigestion and trapped wind.

Other Essential Oils for Weight Loss

Tangerine - A diuretic and is also used to calm the nervous system.
Orange - Helps overcome depression and gives emotional support.
Ylang ylang - Used to clarify thoughts and assist in a feeling of wellness and calm.
Patchouli - Used as a sedative and relaxation aid.

Appendix

Points to avoid on pregnant women

Points whose stimulation sends the vital energy in the lower body, acts on the uterus or the fetus, or strengthens the Yang energy, should not be punctured on a pregnant woman. In addition, do not press heavily on the shoulders.

Three Miles (Stomach 36)

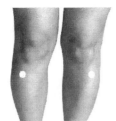

On the outer side of the leg (both right and left legs), 4 finger widths below the knee cap.

Adjoining Valley (Large Intestine 4)

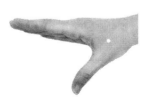

In the webbing between the thumb and index finger.

Three Yin Crossing (Spleen 6)

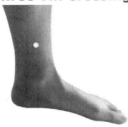

On the inner side of the lower leg, four finger-widths above the anklebone. The point is next to the back of the shinbone.

Big Stream (Kidney 3)

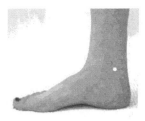

Behind the prominent ankle bone in the depression on the outer side of the ankle. The point is in the hollow between the tip of your ankle bone and the Achilles tendon, on the inner side of the ankle.

Shoulder Well (Gall Bladder 21)

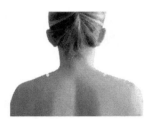

On the thick roll of muscle on top of both shoulders. You will find the point midway between the outer tip of the shoulder and the base of the neck.

Reaching Inside (Bladder 67)

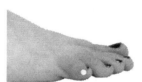

On the outside of the little toe, at the base of the toenail.

About the Author

Hi I am **Anne Cossé**.

I am a Certified Acupressure Practitioner by the USA and France.
I am trained in traditional Shiatsu, Zen Shiatsu, Jin Shin Do, Reflexology, Touch for Health. I am also a Reiki Master & Teacher.

Since 2005 I have practiced therapeutic acupressure in Asia and Europe and delivered self-help acupressure workshops to thousands of people.

One of my thrills is to share my knowledge, whether through my books or via the many media that interviewed me around the world!

**For more TIPS and more TUTORIALS,
visit my websites:**

www.acupressurewellness.com
www.facialacupressure.com
www.youtube.com/annecosse
www.facebook.com/FacialRejuvenationAcupressure
www.pinterest.com/annecosse

Manufactured by Amazon.ca
Bolton, ON